BEAUTY

IS MORE

THAN SKIN DEEP

(Living with Eczema)

By

GwenDolyn Yarborough-Hall

First Edition - First Printing

Copyright © 2008 GwenDolyn Yarborough-Hall. All rights reserved. No part of this book may be reproduced, stored in a retrieval system, or transmitted by any means, electronic, mechanical, photocopying, recording or otherwise, without written permission from the author.

ISBN Number: 978-1-56411-509-6
Library of Congress Control Number: 2008933540

Poem titled "Ron (Gwen Misses You)" written by Leatrice Porcher
All other poems written by GwenDolyn Yarborough-Hall

PRINTED IN THE USA BY:
CB Publishing & Design, LLC
210 East Arrowhead Drive
Charlotte, NC 28213
704.509.2226

Dedication

This book is dedicated to my parents, Virginia "Ms. Daisy" and the spirit of Baxter "Rugged" Yarborough, family, ancestors, friends, students, spiritual guides, teachers and eczema survivors.

9/30/2K8

Thank you Queen Sheana for all you do for us.

Gwen AKA Yuhuna AKA Phyliss

Acknowledgments

Everything that exists is spirit. I thank the God Father/Mother Spirit for using me to tell my-story of being an eczema survivor.
Thanks to my parents and their parents and their parents and all the souls and ancestors that lived.

Thanks to:
My siblings: Ronald, Nancy, Valerie and Kim for their support over the years; my godmother, Shirley Grant, for always encouraging me; to the spirit of my beloved husband, Ronald Hall for introducing me to spirituality and for loving me; friends: Skip, Dorothy, Renee, Joan, Pat Mary, Frank, Mike, Cameron, Darlene, Tanya, Deeborah, Carole, Valdemenia, Priscilla, Renee & Anthony and their daughter, Jasmine,Maria,Phyllis,Yvette and Ann

Thanks to my spiritual leaders and guides:
Rev. Dr. J. Alfred Smith and the Allen Temple family, Oakland, California;Rev. Anne Gehman and the Center for Spiritual Enlightenment, Fairfax, Virginia;Tuesday Spirits Group of Tyson Corner, Virginia and the leaders Vanessa Anseloni, PsyD, PhD and
Daniel Santos, PharmD, PhD www.ssb@ssbaltimore.org

Thanks to those who enhanced my beauty:
Monica R. Maith, MRM Designs, Inc. www.mrmdesignsinc.com
Stras, hair designer Straws289@msn.com
Raymond Henderson, photographer rhendersonphotographer@msn.com

Special thanks to:
Dorothy Walker, Editor
CB Publishing & Design staff
Dr. Joseph Bikowski www.bikowskimd.com and Logical Images at www.Logical Images.com for granting me permission to use their photos.

What is Beauty?

"Beauty is eternity, gazing at itself in a mirror."
Kahlil Gibran

Physical beauty is superficial and is not as important as a person's intellectual, emotional, and spiritual qualities.
The New Dictionary of Cultural Literacy, Third Edition 2002

Table of Contents

Preface

For the majority of my life, I had to deal with the stares, jokes and comments from people who said that I was "ugly" to the bone.

Why was I created with this disease? Why was I teased and stared at all the time? Why was my skin so dark and dry that it resembled an alligator?

These were questions I asked God and my parents every day from the time I was five. I was so tired of itching, scratching and bleeding; and itching and scratching, and bleeding. I remember times my mommy would wrap my hands at night so I would not scratch. My daddy took on extra jobs to pay the medical expenses that were piling up because of my skin condition.

I was told that I was allergic to tomatoes, wool, chocolate, all citrus fruit, the sun, the cold weather and the list goes on and on.

What is Eczema?

Eczema (atopic dermatitis) is a chronic, recurring inflammatory skin disease that is most common in people with a family history of an atopic disorder such as asthma, or hay fever. Eczema is characterized by patchy, dry, itchy and scaly areas of skin. In severe cases of eczema, the skin can weep, bleed, and crust over. Many experts think that eczema occurs when you have an inherited tendency for the disease, and the disease is "triggered." Triggers can vary widely, and some examples are stress, or sensitivity and exposure to certain soaps, fabrics or foods.

The skin is the biggest organ. Living with skin that is damaged and deformed because of eczema and other atopic diseases is emotionally, physically and spiritually draining. Many times I asked myself why was I the one bearing this disease. Now that I am older I see why—so I can be a testimony to others.

What causes eczema? Food, environment, stress and genetics play a big role in getting this disease. I learned recently that there are millions of people on this planet, young and old, from all walks of life who are suffering from eczema.

There is a case of a 70-year-old woman experiencing eczema for the first time in her life. She mentioned that she got this disease near the end of her life because her faith in God made her realize she did not have long to scratch.

In the past, I would tease my parents by telling them that they must have made me in a barn or on some hay because I'm the only one of their children who has this disease. When they made the other children they had a nice comfortable bed. We all would laugh. Yes, laughter is the best medicine.

Images of Eczema

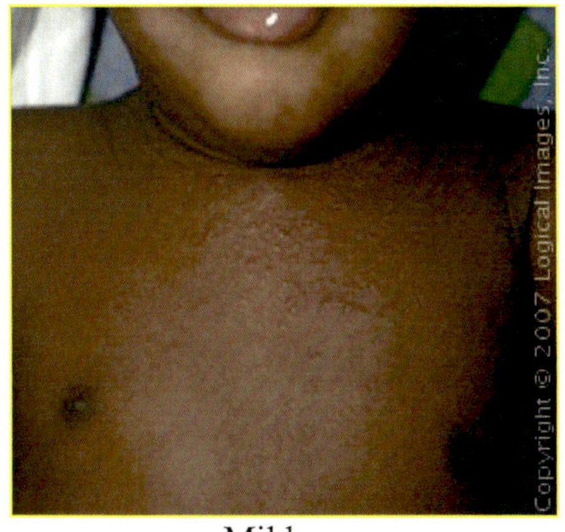

Mild

Used with permission from Logical Images

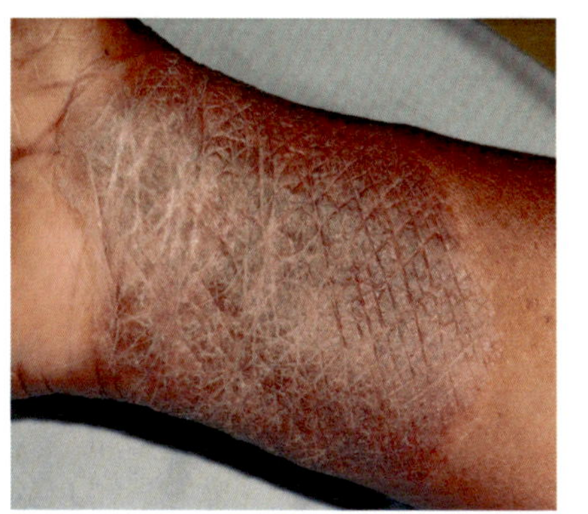

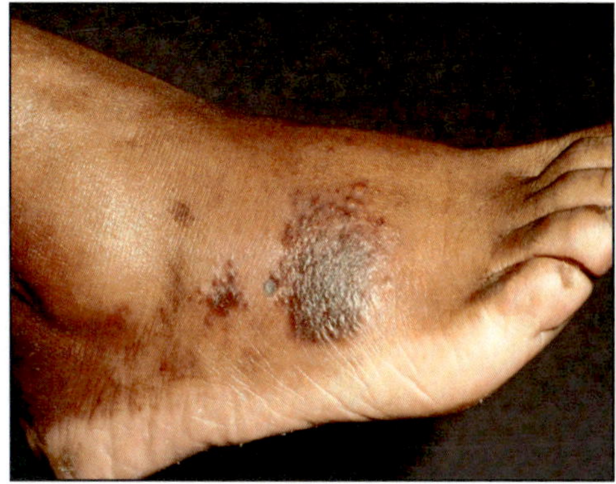

Extreme

arm foot

Used with permission from Dr. Joseph Bikowski

In the Beginning

I am the first of five children born to Virginia "Ms. Daisy" Dunston and Baxter "Rugged" Yarborough. They grew up as next door neighbors in Louisburg, North Carolina.

My father was a proud man who protected and provided for his family. After graduating from Louisburg High School he joined the United States Navy. His tour of duty included being a cook during World War II. He often spoke of the sweltering heat in the Canary Islands near northwest Africa and the insect infested jungles of Burma. I feel that exposure to such environments without proper treatment could have, in some way, contributed to what was passed on to his offspring.

My mother was the oldest of three children who moved to Louisburg with her family after her mother passed away. Her father re-married. He was a minister at several churches within the state of North Carolina. His wife treated his children very badly. I know that my mother felt that marriage would be her only means of escape from the harsh treatment from the "Cinderella stepmother syndrome."

When my parents married, they were headed to New York. My mom told us that she wanted her children to speak the New York dialect. That never happened because they stopped in Washington, DC. Me and all of my siblings were born and raised in southeast in the Anacostia area. We lived in the southeast projects known as Frederick Douglass Dwelling. In the summer of 1963 we moved into our first home in Shipley Terrace. I was in the 9th grade at Frederick Douglass Junior High School.

I remember my first real test of faith at age seven. I attended Emmanuel Baptist Church on Ainger Place, in southeast Washington, DC. The entrance to the main sanctuary included a painting by the late John Robinson, a famous painter. The painting was a picture of a brown-skinned Jesus sitting with outstretched hands. There is an inscription of the words in Matthew 11:28 "Come unto me all ye that are burden and heavy laden take my yolk upon me."

On this particular Sunday, I was really desperate when I entered the main sanctuary. I cried out, "Okay Lord, I'm going to give this burden to You—either You heal my skin or take me on home. I'm tired of the itching, scratching, bleeding and most of all the stares and teasing. Father, please heal me."

I remember reading how Jesus healed the people with leprosy. If He could heal people with leprosy so long ago, why couldn't He heal me,

I wondered? To me eczema was more or less an updated version of leprosy. There was no one I could talk to about what I was feeling or how much I was suffering.

The outbreaks continued. One outbreak in 1960 was so bad I could not participate in my graduation from Stanton Elementary School. My skin looked and felt like it had been burned all over my body, including my face. The outbreak was so bad it developed into impetigo with pus oozing from my scalp, neck, ears—all over my body.

During my freshman year at Douglas Junior High School, I missed 35 days, almost an entire semester, because I was hospitalized due to an outbreak of eczema.

I am terrified of needles even to this day (however, I found out that the butterfly needle does not hurt). I remember the doctor trying to get blood from me. I was so scared I screamed hysterically and broke the needle before the doctor could draw my blood. The broken needle stayed on the floor of the hospital until the next day. My parents were furious when they found out.

In 1963, I was a freshman at Anacostia High School and my skin was a little better. By this time of my life I had really become an introvert, a hermit of sorts. Looking back, I remember getting my first pair of glasses when I was seven years old. It seems that my skin and poor eyesight contributed to me having an inferiority complex.

I was shy and very timid and was terrified when a boy talked to me. I thought he would see my skin and would start teasing me. Actually, the eczema was in remission so I really had nothing to worry about. Yet, I remained self-conscious and I retreated.

I remember reading a lot of books and taking dance lessons. Throughout the Shipley Terrace neighborhood I had the reputation of being a good dancer. When I got up the courage to attend neighborhood parties, I had a good time and didn't really worry about my skin. I just wanted to dance to records by James Brown or the Temptations.

By the time I graduated from high school, I started my first good government job at Federal Communications Commission and began taking college courses and learned as much as I could about computers at Federal City College (now University of the District of Columbia). I had a few outbreaks, but nothing as bad as what I experienced during the early 1960s, so I thought.

Educating an Educator

I guess you could say I was always intrigued with computers. While working at the University of the District of Columbia, I was introduced to my first computer—the IBM Display Writer. This machine consisted of a keyboard with a one line display. The display screen was amber, which was really bad on the eyes. Setting margins and tabs consisted of knowing codes.

While in California, I took courses at various Peralta College campuses. During the summer of 1985, I took a class at California Polytechnic which prepared me academically for my purpose in life—teaching people how to use computers. I obtained a teaching credential and taught my first typing class at a middle school in Oakland, California. I began to market myself and conducted my first bag lunch seminar for executives at a bank in California. The seminar was a success and I realized my gift of making people feel comfortable and confident when using the computer.

I offered a basic computer class at Solano Community College in Suisun City, California that was ranked number one in registration and attendance. The rest is history or "my" story.

As my dearest male friend, Skip Bryant once told me, "Gwen you are something else. You teach at universities, colleges, military institutions and the list goes on and on, and you do not have a college degree." I said, "Skip, I do have one degree, but teaching is my purpose and gift in this life."

I attended University of the District of Columbia, California Polytechnic, Peralta Colleges in Oakland, California, J Sargeant Reynolds in Richmond, Virginia (where I earned my Associates Degree in Office Systems Technology), Old Dominion University, Norfolk, Virginia and Department of Defense Information School, Ft.Meade, Maryland.

I have and continue to fulfill my gift from God by providing computer instruction at a number of places including Virginia State University, Petersburg, Virginia; Prince George's Community College, Largo, Maryland; J Sargeant Reynolds Community College, Richmond, Virginia; Department of Justice, Philip Morris, Arbitron, Lucent Technology, Museum of Virginia and Nabisco Foods.

I taught classes at J Sargeant Reynolds during the day and took classes at night or on the weekends at Old Dominion University. When I moved back to the DC area in 2002 I went to the University of the District of Columbia to find out if my life experience and credits would afford me the opportunity to graduate. I was told that I had duplicate classes. I came home with tears in my eyes—another obstacle to prevent me from obtaining another degree. I lit candles and began to meditate. It was during my periods of meditation that it was revealed to me that teaching was my gift despite society's notion that I needed a degree.

I am an educator. My purpose is to teach. I followed numerous paths to educate myself and in doing so, I am fulfilling my dream of educating others. I've been teaching for over 20 years and received numerous awards, including Who's Who Among America's Teachers on four occasions; and I have Microsoft certification.

Spirituality

I remember during my summer visits to my grandparents in Louisburg, North Carolina, I'd have severe outbreaks. It could be 90° outside, yet I would wear long sleeved blouses and long pants because I was embarrassed by the stares and snickering people made towards me when they saw my rough, dry, broken skin. I remember sitting on the front porch at night, staring at what I thought were millions of stars in the sky, wondering and asking God what was my purpose; would I be cured of this disease, would I ever find happiness; and thousands of other questions.

During those quiet times of looking at the night sky, I knew that there was a source/power/spirit greater than myself. I marveled at the beauty of the stars and used them as the focal point of communicating with my Creator. I guess you could say that was the beginning of my spiritual journey. During one session of sitting on the porch, I had a vision of a young man, brown complexion, elongated face. How was I supposed to know that this man in my vision was destined to be my husband?

On Memorial Day 1966 I met a young man who would change my life forever. This is the same man that I saw in a vision when I was a young girl staring at the stars from my Yarborough grandparents' front porch. This young man gave me encouragement and saw beauty in me. He saw that my spirit and soul were beautiful and that my skin was radiant. He taught me about spiritualism and unconditional love. He told me never to change my personality and to keep a positive attitude. That man was Ronald E. Hall, born in Rock Hill, South Carolina, raised in Shirlington, Virginia. We were married for three fantastic, short years. We lived in Fairfax, Virginia.

Ronald taught me about spiritualism. He often mentioned how much he loved me and that he would always love me. He shared scripture and affirmations for me to repeat daily. I remember him telling me that he could do more for me in the "spirit world" than he could in the physical world. At the time I did not understand to what he was referring. Now I know.

My life as Mrs. Ronald E. Hall was an adventure of love and devotion. There were many times when I received unexpected gifts of lingerie, flowers, and outfits—just because he loved me. I remember us going on several mini vacations at the spur of the moment. One was our trip to visit my maternal great-aunt, Mae Underwood, in New York. I learned a lot about life from my maternal aunt Mae. We also visited Ronnie's best friend, Ronnie Knotts. We visited our grandmothers in North Carolina and South Carolina.

Even when we went grocery shopping it was an adventure. After Ronald passed, I found it difficult to go grocery shopping for a long time, but I had to eat right—yes, I adjusted. Losing the only man that really, truly loved me was a horrible experience. It seemed our life as one was just beginning and suddenly it was gone. This emotional trauma due to the loss drove me to an outbreak.

Earlier I mentioned that I felt I was on a spiritual journey. I was raised as a Baptist. When I lived in California I became a deaconess at Allen Temple Baptist Church and started a litigural dance ministry, which was unheard of at that time. I remember several of the elderly deaconesses referring to me as the "dancing deaconess." My first performance was at a singles retreat cruise on the San Francisco Bay. I danced to the Lord's Prayer, sung by Johnny Mathis and Gladys Knight. The audience was very ecstatic and accommodating. They had never experienced such a performance. I began to get invitations to dance at various churches throughout California.

When I became a deaconess I felt very proud because I was the only granddaughter following in the footsteps of grandmother Nancy

Yarborough. The pilgrimage to the Holy Land with Allen Temple members heightened my spiritual curiosity.

When I moved to Richmond, Virginia I became a deaconess at First Baptist Church. I was often referred to as the "sassy" deaconess because I did not fit the model of being the traditional married woman with children. Yes, I was lively for my Creator.

When I moved back to DC in 2002 I inquired about becoming a deaconess at Emmanuel Baptist Church, the church I attended as a child. I was told I had "to be married to a deacon." My response was who is going to minister to the single and widows of the church? That was it! I'd had enough of traditional, organized religion.

I began to meditate and read books by Deepak Chopra, Wayne Dwyer, Edgar Cayce, Gary Zukav and others. I learned that this body is temporary and that my soul spirit will return to the source, "The Creator/Infinite Intelligence/God/Goddess," when I have learned all the lessons destined for me. I've learned to listen to my spirit guides and call on the thousands of angels that are always with me.

While teaching a class at the Department of Justice, Criminal Division, I met Tanya "Stras" Smith. Stras and I began to talk. We learned that we both had lost a loved one—me a husband and her a son. That was the beginning of a very spiritual relationship. She introduced me to the

Center of Spiritual Enlightenment in Fairfax, Virginia. We both became members in September 2007. I have learned so much about life and the transition process. Yes, we are only pilgrims passing through time and space on planet Earth.

Migration

It seems that every decade I move somewhere. During the 1970s I lived in northern Virginia as a newlywed. I lived in northern California during the 1980s as a widow. In the 1990s I moved to central Virginia to be closer to my parents who lived in Washington, DC. It is now a new millennium and I'm writing this while living in Maryland. Who knows where I will eventually live—hopefully, somewhere it doesn't snow.

During the migrations I've met people who are still near and dear to me. While living in northern Virginia, I met Shirley Yorker, who was my next door neighbor. Shirley was given the talent of being an extraordinary seamstress. When I moved back to the DC metro area in 2002, we continued our friendship. She still sews and is constantly making monogrammed gifts or altering ethnic clothes for me. Thank you Shirley.

California

I knew that one day I wanted to live in California. I did not realize while being married, that I had to lose in order to gain. My loss was when I became a widow in 1979. My gain was when I moved to northern California in 1980.

The eczema was in a dormant state from 1980 until about 1983. In 1984 my skin began to break out occasionally. During this time, I had the opportunity to go on a pilgrimage to the Holy Land led by Rev. J. Alfred Smith, Jr., pastor of Allen Temple Baptist Church in Oakland, California. While there I bottled water from the Dead Sea and applied it to my skin which cleared it up immediately. Finally, I thought I am healed!

While in California I met some wonderful friends and associates. My first friend was Theodore Mike Casey, who was in the transportation business. In fact his family business moved my household goods from Alexandria, Virginia to Alameda, California. Mike showed me around and introduced me to his family and close friends.

Later I met Dorothy Walker, who was my supervisor when we worked at Safeway Stores, Incorporated in Oakland, California. Dorothy attended Howard University. We immediately became friends because of the DC bond. Later we found out that my younger sister was marrying her cousin. While attending a professional organizational meeting in San

Francisco I met Renee Richardson. We were the only two women of color at the Women in Telecommunications meeting, San Francisco chapter. We later learned that we both attended the same church, Allen Temple. I became very active at Allen Temple and met a lot of people including Mary Amos, who affectionately calls me Onion Head and Pat Dunson who became my first client when I launched my computer business.

During my time in California my creative side really developed. I began to write poetry as a means of getting through the grieving process. I became a member of the Widows Network-the youngest and only woman of color.

I began to recite my poems in churches and at various events including the Juneteenth Festival in San Jose and for the Bay Area Black Journalist awards ceremony. My close friends told me my poems were good. However, it wasn't until I recited poems at the Bay Area Black Journalist Association and received a standing ovation that I really knew people appreciated what I had to say. I was so in awe when I saw the audience standing and cheering I thought to myself, "why are these people standing up." Then I realized—they were standing up and applauding me. I continued writing poetry and entering my poems into contests. I submitted my poems to the local Alameda, California newspaper. One

Saturday while shopping, I purchased a newspaper and to my surprise and amazement I saw my poems in print. I was so excited.

I was also involved with the Black Filmmakers Hall of Fame, which is equivalent to the Academy Awards. I wrote articles about the Black Filmmakers and got a chance to meet several cast members who performed in the movie, ***The Color Purple***.

I received an unexpected award for my poetry from the San Francisco Chapter of the Black Chamber of Commerce. I do not write poems now as much as I did while living in California.

Living on the west coast was definitely good for my soul, spirit and body. Later, I met another poet, Joan Geurin. I've learned that God uses me as a catalyst of bonding people. I introduced Dorothy, Renee and Joan to each other. We became good friends and remain close to this day.

I was always very ambitious and as my Aunt Jo always told me, "I did it my way." I remember going to a temporary agency to sign up for work when I first moved to California. The counselor asked me if I knew how to use an IBM computer. I said yes. When I left the agency I noticed the IBM store was on the corner. I went in and tinkered with the IBM PC until I found the on/off switch and practiced creating documents for about 10 minutes. I then felt that I was ready for any job that required knowledge of a computer. I was so proud of myself and got a job as a word processor at Safeway Stores, Incorporated and later at the San Francisco Foundation.

I moved to Suisun, California in the mid 1980s. I started working as a computer instructor at Travis AFB and became the first female board member for the local computer club. I met Deeborah Webster who was in the military while working at Travis AFB. She was in my first class at the base and we became good friends. Who would have known that decades later we would renew our friendship in 2007 in Maryland.

Richmond; Virginia

My parents were getting older and the impact of the 1989 Bay Area earthquake were the reasons I moved back to the east coast, this time Richmond, Virginia in the early 1990s. Once I moved back to the east coast, eczema outbreaks began again. I went to dermatologists in Richmond only to be told that my skin disease was heredity and I would always have it. This time the outbreaks were especially bad on my neck, back, and ankles. Once the outbreak on my back was in the shape of a Christmas tree. I later learned that was an outbreak of pityriasis, another skin condition marked by dry scaly patches of skin. It was difficult for me to apply the medication to my back.

One outbreak was so terrible I was in tears when I called my parents in Washington, DC. My dad told me he was so sorry I had to suffer. He had been diagnosed with shingles and sent me some of his medicine. During this outbreak, I thought about Job and how he lost everything—children, land, friends. His skin broke out really bad and yet he trusted and had faith in God. God restored everything to Job that he lost and healed his body from the terrible sores. Why, I thought didn't God do the same for me?

I remember my first day walking into the computer lab at J. Sargent Reynolds College. One of the students, Andréa Baker Barnes Johnson, who I later befriended, was so loud that day announcing with pride that "we have a Black woman as our computer instructor who is dressed in a nice navy blue suit and is willing to share her knowledge with us." Andréa followed, no, she exceeded me. She is presently teaching in the public school system in Washington, DC.

I met other people while teaching in Richmond who are very dear to me. There is Cameron Hardison who I met when I was a contractor at AT&T (aka Lucent Technology). We found out that our relatives knew each other (my dad and her uncle). It seemed as if it was destined that we meet.

Another student was Darlene Chinn. I often referred to Darlene as my "worst" student simply because she would want my attention with a problem right away. It did not matter that I had just helped her two minutes before. When I moved to Maryland, Darlene was my first visitor. She calls me her mentor.

I met Jan Robinson, who is an ardent car collector. While attending a motorcycle affair in Richmond we met and learned that we were both raised in southeast Washington, DC. Jan and I would drive to DC just to attend a nice dance party. He was always available when I had problems with my car.

Kenny Griffin, affectionately known as Kenny G, was my number one supporter. We met at church and became good friends. Kenny would check on me when I had outbreaks and would even play his doctor role. He put on plastic gloves to apply topical medicines on my back, which was a great help since there were areas I could not reach. Thank you Kenny.

Another friend, JW Harris, was a widower with children and grandchildren. We became good friends because we could both relate to losing a spouse and suffering through our bouts with skin ailments. JW had psoriasis.

After my daddy passed in 2001, I moved back to the DC area to be with my mom. I began to have severe outbreaks on my neck, arms and even nipples. I went to several dermatologists in the area who prescribed various steroidal creams which I did not want to use for fear of the side effects. The side effects include: high blood pressure and heart disease, liver damage, cancer, stroke, blood clots, urinary and bowel problems, and other more severe illnesses.

Relief

In July 2006 during a severe outbreak, I was referred to Dr. James Daile, a naturopath, by my sister, Valerie, who is a survivor of Scleroderma, a disease that affects the immune system. Dr. Daile performed a test on me that is administered to astronauts before they travel in space. I call it the "21st century physical." No blood is drawn and no needles are used. Water is applied to the index finger which is linked to a computer program. As a result of that test, I found out I was allergic to catfish, flounder, lima beans, grits, corn (including popcorn), yeast, bananas, eggs, milk, cheese, and crabs. These are foods I ate religiously every day for years. This was the first time I was ever tested to learn of my foods allergies. I started eliminating those foods from my diet and went on a detoxification regime eating yams, almonds, avocado and drinking lots of water. I began wearing a detoxifying patch every other day. In about three weeks I started seeing results. My skin was clearing up and I was losing weight. I went from a size 14 petite to a size 10.

I also learned about DermaTechRx, a Q-based company that manufactures products to bring relief to eczema suffers. I spoke to the president, Sandra Booher, who sent me complimentary care packages of ointments, Dead Sea salts, and body washes. Using the products and eliminating certain foods from my diet cleared up my skin tremendously. Now when I receive calls from desperate eczema suffers, I refer them to DermaTechRx so that they can receive their care packages. I also started using a natural soap created by Dawn Worthy, whose son Elias has been suffering with eczema since he was two years of age. Dawn used all natural ingredients to create a soap that finally bought Elias some relief.

In August 2006, I went on a mini-retreat with high school classmates (Diane Hood, Clavon Kinard, Billie Amos and JoAnn Murray) to Colonial Beach, Virginia, the summer home of JoAnn Murray. We were excited about getting away and eating crabs. Well, I was not able to eat crabs, but I could eat salmon. The "girls," as Diane's granddaughter affectionately calls us, were so very supportive. I must say during my ordeal with this disease I've had a great support system of family, friends, associates and students.

In April 2007 I went to my primary physician, Dr. Lynn Yarborough (yes, my cousin). She said, " Cuz, never let your skin get this bad before you seek help." She gave me a shot of steroids which helped a lot and I did not experience any side effects. In the summer of 2007 my skin was looking good. In July, I attended the National Eczema Association's Conference in Crystal City, Virginia. There were over 1400 eczema survivors in attendance, including adults and children. There were two attendees from England and Brazil. We had a great time sharing the trials and tribulations of dealing with eczema. Children were so excited that they could wear shorts without worrying about people staring at the outbreaks of eczema on their legs.

After having such a good time, I noticed my neck was breaking out from wearing the badge at the convention. During one of the sessions we learned to soak our bodies in a cupful of Clorox along with Dead Sea salts. This remedy helped a little. I still had signs of an outbreak but not as bad as it was in July.

In August the outbreak began to get worse. During this time I was breaking out on my left leg, arms and breast. I was itching, scratching and bleeding especially at night. I was unable to sleep because of the discomfort. I was absent from work at least one day per week from September to October due to the outbreak.

Working in an office at Andrews AFB with over 20 people (each person having at least three computers) did not help much since the equipment generated so much heat. The room was not designed to accommodate all the heat even though two makeshift air conditioners were put in the room. I could not wait until my eight-hour work day was over so I could disrobe from all of my clothing.

In August 2007 I received a massage from Kathy English Holt, who is also a survivor of eczema. She noticed the outbreak on the left side of my body—arm, back and behind the knee. I learned from Kathy that the left side of the body deals with maternal instincts, caring about others. She asked if I was worried about my mother. I did not think I was worried about anyone, but I guess subconsciously I was concerned because my sister, Valerie, needs a lung transplant and my mother has dementia and needs to be relocated to Maryland (both are presently living in Washington State).

I went to cousin Dr. Lynn in October. This time she prescribed Singular and Zrytec to be taken orally once a day. So far, so good. I'm getting compliments on how my skin is glowing. I started using black soap and shea butter along with Vaseline®.

National Eczema Association

While surfing the Internet one day, I found the National Eczema Association, based in Marin County, California. I contacted them and completed an application to become a group leader. I felt it was my purpose to connect with children and adults who are living with eczema. Once I became a group leader, I began to get phone calls and emails from all over the world. Some of the calls and emails included:

- An uncle whose two-month old niece living in India was diagnosed with eczema. He was crying out for help. Should the mother move to the United States? Should they stay in India? He had questions I could not answer. I asked questions about the mother's diet and if she was breast feeding the young baby.
- An adult male who had to leave his teaching job in Las Vegas and move to Indiana because of eczema. He was heartbroken

and there was a severe outbreak on his face. He was a middle school teacher and had to contend with his students making fun of him. I encouraged him to contact a dermatologist in his area, refrain from drinking sodas and start drinking lots of water.

- Iris, an older woman in Washington, DC who had not been out of her apartment since January 2006. She began to develop bed sores.
- A mother who has an 11-year-old daughter who cannot attend school because her skin is badly infected with eczema. When I read her email, tears and feelings from my early years of suffering with eczema surfaced again.

I am encouraging many people who are seeking help from this disease. Mothers are thanking me. Children are thanking me. I am thanking my Creator for using me to tell my story to provide a source of relief for the survivors.

I have truly come to accept that "coincidence is God's way of being anonymous." Well that certainly is what happened when I met Renee Dantzler, mother of Jasmine, an eczema survivor. Richard Cox, co-worker at Andrews AFB, told me about one of his church members whose daughter's experience with eczema was published in a community newspaper. He gave me the mother's email address and we began to communicate. Renee Dantzler is a very strong, determined mother seeking relief for her daughter.

The first meeting of the DC Metropolitan chapter of the National Eczema Association was held on December 30, 2006 at the Clinton, Maryland library. It was so uplifting to finally meet Renee and Jasmine. Others in attendance included a mother and her son, a mother seeking information for her daughter, a young man around 20 years old and a young woman who stopped simply because she saw the sign on the blackboard. Each of us was relieved to finally be able to speak to others who were going through the same bout with eczema and all its symptoms.

Hope

It is spring 2008. My skin is breaking out on the back of my arms, bend of legs and this time on my face including the skin around both eyes. I am constantly wiping tears from both eyes and trying not to scratch.

In reflecting over my life with this disease, I now know why my Creator used me to share my testimony of being a survivor on this journey. There may not be a cure for this disease in my lifetime. I will continue to try ointments, soak in a capful of Clorox for a few moments or anything else that relieves the itch including meditating and seeing and feeling my skin as clear and not itching.

Beauty is more than skin deep. Beauty for me has emerged through my spirit, determination, hope and support from those I've met along the way. I pray that some of the words in this book will bring a sense of hope, comfort and determination to those who are living with eczema.

Reflections from My Family

Sister, Valerie Yarborough

"All I remember is that you were miserable. You scratched and shit a lot. You would make that noise as you tried to get some ease to your inner torture. You were introverted and stayed to yourself a lot. You could not do anything. Some things were to your advantage as you could not wash dishes, you could not wash clothes, you could not wear wool (that wasn't good because it was cold). You could not stay outside long. You were always haunted by the childhood taunting of your peers, they called you rashy tashy and that hurt you so much. I felt sorry for you but when it came to the dishes, huh! you got over like a fat rat. I am glad that you finally have some relief and are doing well and helping others to heal. Keep up the good work."

Cousin, Rosetta Yarborough Terry

"The only place I can remember you having eczema was right under your nose in the summer."

Aunt Nan Dunston

"I remembered that you had a very difficult time with the eczema but did not remember that much about it. I do remember how your skin looked so rough, that you had a lot of itching and how it was just cumbersome. To be honest with you I had forgotten that you ever had the disease."

Sister, Nancy Yarborough Thorpe

"What I remember the most was that when you got a bad breakout you felt really bad. You thought you looked really bad but actually, you didn't. You were my sister and I wanted to comfort you and let you know it was okay, but, you were the oldest and for some reason I thought because you were older, it didn't count what I thought."

Aunt Mamie Dunston Hall

Poem

S SEE
Skin is here for ever
Eczema was not to the bone
Eczema faded away but my beautiful skin has
held it's own

K Kiss me and do not fear

I In God I trusted

N Now I'm Healed

© 2008 Mamie Dunston Hall

Aunt Jamel Covington Taborn

"My earliest introduction to your eczema was my first summer on a visit to Aunt Virginia-bread and Uncle Rugged's home. Your eyes were very red, weeping, and swollen. Your neck was flared, with patches of superficial openings and weeping. I checked your meds and you were taking the Prednisone taper, Benadryl, and Periactin for the itching. The saddest restriction I remember was that everyone was going out for ice cream, and you were not allowed outside due to the hot weather. I also remember that the house was hotter than the outdoors. We did not have air conditioning, but you were allowed to use the big old dusty fan, blowing hot air. I also remember the wise words from your mother, "You think

Gwen's skin is bad, you should have seen her before I took her to the doctor."

Brother, Ronald Yarborough

“I often prayed that God would take the disease from you and give it to me because I felt I could deal with the teasing better than you. I remember some of the medicine you had to put on was stinky. You had to endure the pain and the unpleasant smell.”

Cousin, Cathy Yarborough

“I'm giving the short version of the childhood I remember. When we were children in North Carolina, you had a rash. I didn’t know or understand at the time what was wrong with your skin. I just knew that you had a rash. You would whine and scratch a lot. You wouldn't come outside much, if at all. When Ronald and I would be outside playing in the yard you would stay inside the whole day. You didn't like bugs, or the sun. Aunt Mary wanted to take us fishing or to pick berries, or get pecans out of the tree, and all of the cousins went except you. You stayed in the house. Grandma Yarborough would put creams on you. I felt so bad for you with that dark rash over your body. You and cousin Sheila both had rash all over your bodies. I would feel so bad for you. I wanted to do something for you but didn't know what was wrong except that you were miserable.

Now, I'm older and know. I had my own dealings with this disease first- hand because my own baby and last child suffered from eczema."

Photos

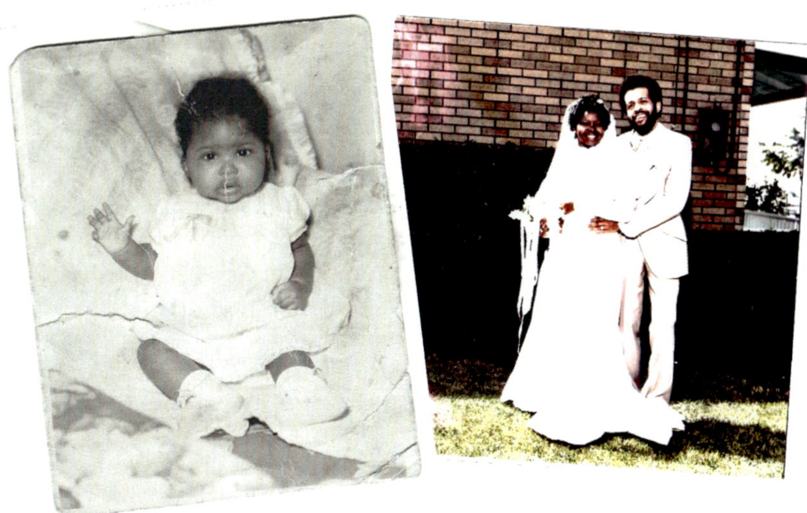

6 months old

Wedding photo
June 5, 1976

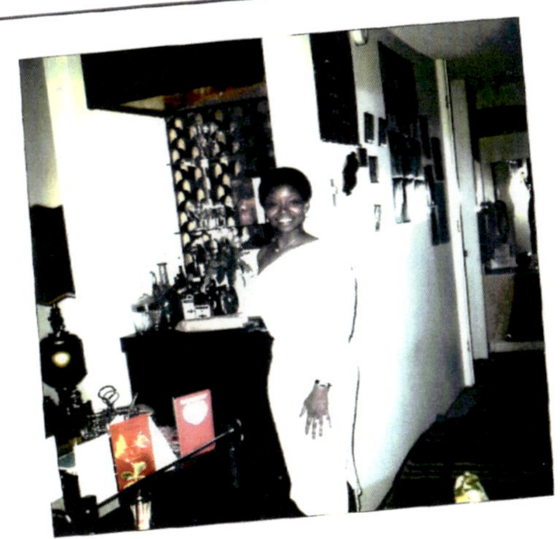

February 1985
Alameda, CA

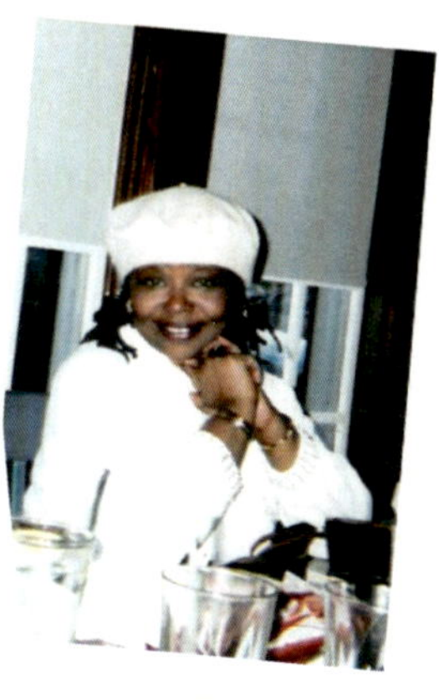

January 2003
Temple Hills, MD

Litany of Poems

RON (GWEN MISSES YOU)

Dedicated to GwenDolyn from former student

Ron, my arms miss you
my hands miss you,
my fingers and thumbs miss you.
My eyes miss your lips as you speak
my ears miss hearing you peacefully asleep,
Ron, my breasts miss you
my stomach too
the round of my hips and my thighs miss you,
my knees miss your tender touch
my calves miss you twice as much
my feet miss you
my toes miss you
but most of all, Ron
My heart misses you

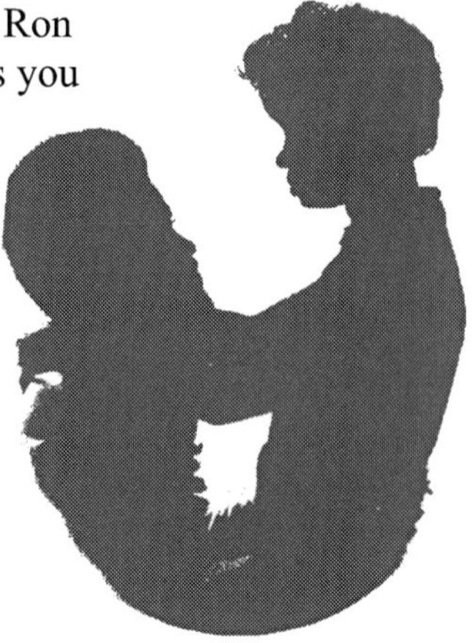

© 1979 LEATRICE PORCHER

WIDOW

WIDOW——EMPTY
WIDOW——WITHOUT SPOUSE
No one to love you, caress and cuddle you
No one to cook for, shop with, make love with
No one to miss you, kiss you, befriend you
No one to share with, balance the checkbook with, play games with
No one to cry with, disagree with, smile with
No one to hold your hand or wash the leftover frying pan
No one to vacation with, attend concerts, church or plays with
No one to escort you to dances, company affairs, or to the movies
No one to prepare snow cream for, or play in the snow with
all these events and more leave an empty feeling within when you become a widow
You ask, dear Lord, why me——why are you leaving me empty?
Years go by before you realize that you were chosen to be an example for other women who become widows
chosen because you are strong and will survive
chosen because you now have to work a 9 to 5
chosen because you are special and will endure
the perils of widowhood and much more!!!!!

CYA

Cover your assets, no one else will
Cover your assets from the enemy
Know who you are and be proud
Hold your head up high and strut with dignity and pride

OVERCOMING FEAR

She was scared, alone and depressed
suddenly, her guardian angel appeared,
"You will have nothing to fear——you are an element of the most high—
you will succeed.
You've passed the test of survival and determination. Your rewards will be many!
They wanted you to fail, fall down to the pits of disgrace and deprivation, but no. You climbed each step——one at a time, tripping occasionally, but never did you stop climbing!
Through faith you will reach the impossible goal——hold on little one for time is beside you, fear is behind you and success in front of you.
Walk proud black pearl."

PEACE

JUST AS A LEAF IS AN EXTENSION OF A TREE;
SO WE ARE AS PEOPLE, AN EXTENSION OF LOVE, HOPE AND PEACE

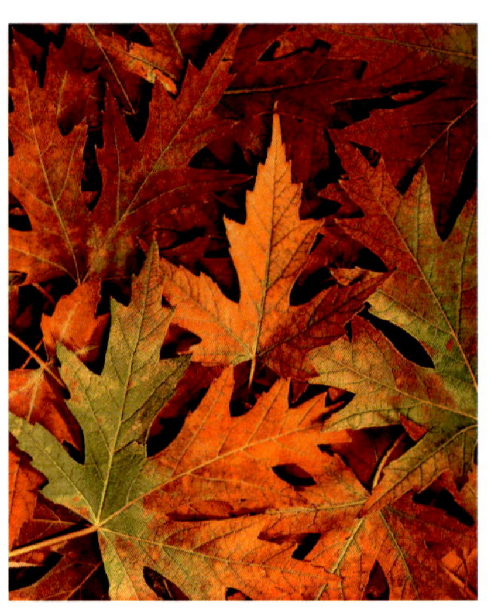

THE BOND

From the time that a sperm attaches itself to an egg
a bond is formed
From the time the umbilical cord is cut from the mother a bond is formed
Through the escapades of childhood into adolescence a bond is formed
From the experiences of adulthood encompassing all that it offers
a bond is formed
That bond will not be broken by any obstacles,
be it marriage, death, or disappointments that
may enter one's life
from that bond, other bonds develop, stronger, but a
bond will never be broken

DETERMINATION

Determination motivates
Fear stagnates
Faith guides
Hope sustains
Love conquers

The Musical Angel

Silence—a genius is approaching the stage. When he struts his long, lean physique across the stage there is silence in the air. He demands and gets the utmost respect.

Some say he was a local boy who made good. I say he was a musical angel obeying the wishes and commands of his Creator.

With the mere flicker of his wrist he made instruments speak the universal language that is understood by all mankind. The trumpets soared to their very highest notes. The violins left an elevating feeling of heavenly, peaceful, harmony deep in my soul. The percussions do not miss a beat when this Maestro conducts.

He showed me some of his favorite places behind the scenes and introduced me to some of the most prestigious musicians in the world.

Music is the universal language that binds mankind without being subjected to the diseases of racism and prejudice.

His music causes halos to float around my environment leaving a soothing remedy for my soul.

The Musical Angel was Calvin Simmons, a model of Black Excellence in the 20th century.

FALLING INTO WINTER

During the fall, the earth goes through myriad changes of
temperature, climatical conditions, environmental and physical
transformations, so does my life!

During the fall I go through changes, affecting my environmental and
physical conditions
The fall season is a time for preparing for the winter, summer and spring
of the coming year

It is a good time to sow deeds of creativity, positivity and productivity
The cold, windy, dark nights to come will be opportunities or me
to utilize the energy I received from the many, sunny, warm days
of summer past

Just as the leaves begin to transform from green into shades of rust, brown
and red
I will transform my thoughts into illuminating
spheres of conquering obstacles to come

FRIENDSHIP

If I could be your friend for a minute, a second during
this journey of life,
I would comfort you through your sorrow, laugh with you at your jokes
hold you to get strength, kiss you to feel love
smile at you to lift your spirits
and befriend you forever

Sensuous Lady

Sensuous lady desired by men skin as soft as cotton
Eyes that dance while flirting with your manhood
beckoning you to come share your love, warmth, body and mind
Luscious lips that will engulf yours like a fluffy pillow
Firm hips that will wrap around your physique, cradling and nurturing your ego…
Let me
Be your
Sensuous lady

Education

If it were not for education, where would you be? Perhaps on Masta Washington's plantation sharecropping
If it were not for education, how would you be able to communicate your hopes, desires and dreams into realities?
Only a few centuries ago, people were denied the liberties of learning
Yet, their hearts and souls were burning and yearning for the knowledge to succeed and eventually surpass college. Well, those dreams have become real
However, there are still some who would rather steal
Education is the key that will unlock many doors so that you can explore
All of the elements and knowledge of this world and much, much more
If it were not for education, where would you be? Perhaps still on Masta Washington's plantation sharecropping
Continue your education for the success of yourself and your nation

The Disappearing Man

The mentality of a man is so frequently hard to understand
His actions and deeds arise out of his own selfish needs.
He has no tact, or respect, for if he did, he would not have just disappeared.
His mother taught him to be courteous and respectful—but what happens to those teachings once he becomes a man?
I do not know, because once he becomes a man, he is so very hard to understand
You show him compassion and share some of your goals
You inquire about his family and peers and listen to him talk about his fears
After giving all of that and more, why---he just disappears
Be careful women for the man is hard to understand
He thinks he is God's gift to sisters all over this land
Respect and dignity---such tiny things to ask

Single

Single—only one
God—only one
Being single sometimes causes me to mingle
with the big boys and men, learning from them all that I possibly can

There are times I hate being single, being only one
No one to come home to after I've worked all day
No one to give me a big hug or kiss my troubles away

When I get like that I look up at the sky
and remember that my Lord, God, is always nearby

We have quiet dates, walking along the beach
We have solitude, peace and quiet
On the days when I cook, He does not require a special diet

So, the times when I feel lonely and feel like I am one
I look up at the stars, moon and sun
I think it is not all that bad, because unlike other singles
I have God as my secret better half

In Our Lifetime

Our lifetime, it was a perplexing time when men were surrounded by computers and phone calls were no longer a dime
In our lifetime, the Bible is being fulfilled—just look around you to see how mankind is going downhill
Fathers killing sons and parents abusing their offspring
How far is man going to continue doing his own thing?

In our lifetime the warnings are being revealed that this capitalistic society is rapidly going down a very destructive hill

Just look around and see how many young girls are actually not even taking the pill

In our lifetime we must become the progressive generation—we must put God first in our quest to become #1 in this nation

Now, let us stop tripping on this negative behavior and start trusting in the Lord, Jesus Christ, our Everlasting Savior

In our lifetime we must strive to be servants of the Master, because our time is running out and His time is approaching must faster.

So, let us stop for a moment in our lifetime and reflect on these little things in life, like love, concern and respect.

THE GIFT

You are a star among many in the galaxy
your leadership and dedication will enable
you to fulfill your goals and desires
You've been the giver most of your life——giving to this one and that
one, but rarely receiving,
now, it is your turn to receive another gift from the creator,
now, don't be afraid or hesitant
for I am your gift!
I will not tarnish, but forever shine like gold
I will not smother you, but will give you space in the universe to grow
spiritually, mentally and physically.
A gift is a token of love from the Creator
Accept it, love it and respect it
before it is gone forever!

What Happens?

What happens when you die?
Why do your survivors cry?
Are you greeted by those ancestors you love?
Do they see your spirit fly like a dove?
Will you remember your days on earth?
Will you travel to another planet of birth?
What happens?

Resources

Dr. Lynn Yarborough
Family Practice and Wellness Consultant
2905 Mitchellville Road, Suite 106
Bowie, MD 20716
301-218-8700

Sandra Booher, Vice President
Dermatechex
info@qbased.com

National Eczema Association
4460 Redwood Highway, Suite 16D
San Rafael, CA 94903
800-818-7546 or 415-499-3474
www.nationaleczema.org

Kathy English Holt, NCTMB
Certified Therapeutic Massage
202-986-1837
kenglishholt@msn.com

Coy Dunston, President
Secrets of Nature (SON)
3923 South Capitol Street, S.W.
Washington, DC 20032

DawnWorthy
dawn@FreshFromtheFarm.Us